Super Detox Diet For Weight Loss

Optimize Your Body's Natural Functions To Detox And
Cleanse Your Body,

Boost Your Health And Lose Weight Naturally.

Eric Warren

CONTENTS

Acknowledgments   i

1   Introduction   1

2   Chapter 1 – WHAT THE OTHER DETOX   3
PROGRAMS PROMISE

3   Chapter 2 – WHAT THE OPTIMUM APPROACH TO   5
DETOX DIET SHOULD BE

4   Chapter 3 – SO WHAT'S TRUE DETOX DIET IS…?   7

5   Chapter 4 – WHAT WE ARE REALLY?   8

6   Chapter 5 – WHAT YOU DON'T UNDERSTAND   9
ABOUT BODY DETOX

7   Chapter 6 – WHAT WE SHOULD BE EATING   12

8   Chapter 7 – ARE THERE ANY ALLOWABLE FATS?   22

9   Chapter 8 – ARE THERE ANY EXCEPTIONS OR   23
SUBSTITUTIONS?

10   Chapter 9 – WILL I EXPERIENCE ANY ADVERSE   24
SYMPTOMS OR EFFECTS?

11   Chapter 10 – WHAT ARE THE CHEATIES   26
AVAILABLE?

12   Chapter 11 – IS EXERCISING REQUIRED?   27

13   Chapter 12 – HOW SHOULD I TRANSITION TO THE   28
DIET 54321?

14   Conclusion   32

15   About The Author   33

ACKNOWLEDGMENTS

The author wishes to thank several people. I would like to thank my wife, Eveline, for her love, support and patience during the past five or so years it has taken me to graduate. I would like to thank my parents for their unending love and support. Last but not least, I would like to thank Edgepedia Publishing, Inc. and my manager John Echols for allowing me to use this subject for my manuscript.

INTRODUCTION

Congratulations! You are on your first step to living a healthier life! Before I divulge everything you need to know about detoxifying your body, here's a disclaimer.

DISCLAIMER

Any and all the contents of this book are based upon the research and opinions of the author, Harold R. Hargreaves, unless otherwise specified.

All the information contained in here does not resolutely aim to replace the information that a qualified healthcare provider offers. Contents must not be regarded as medical advice. The author only intends to share valuable insights and information to the best of his knowledge and research.

The author encourages its readers to conduct own research and make own decision regarding one's health in lieu with the care and guidance of the healthcare providers. Your respective healthcare providers should be aware of your diet and the changes required to such.

Specifically, pregnant and nursing women must consult their physicians before making any changes to their diet.

The book mentions such words as 'cure', 'curing', 'heal', 'healing', etc. These words refer to self-curing and self-healing.

As a Natural Health Coach, the goal of the author is to write and share with his readers the true and natural approaches recognized in healing oneself.

As individuals with different health conditions and diet requirements, there will be discrepancies in results between two individuals who chose to apply their learning from this book. Outcomes can be also influenced by external factors.

By continue reading this book, it means you agree to the conditions noted above.

In lieu with the conditions above, I should include a disclaimer for those under the care and supervision of a physician. Most healthcare providers shun the idea of organic health products and detox. Your clinician may deter you from following the program discussed in here.

Let him/her know that you will follow the program. However, ask him/her that you would appreciate it if s/he will monitor your progress health-wise. If s/he is not open and willing to do so, you may have the option to change your physician with a natural health advisor (naturopath). Nonetheless, if changing your physician is not an option, s/he may be open to the idea of working with a naturopath.

The detox diet that I am going to teach you may go against everything you know about losing weight naturally and specifically, healthy eating. The diet changes may be even drastic. Rest assured, however, that the program is both safe and effective. You will lose weight the way you want and achieve a healthier mind and body in the process.

Enjoy your detox journey!

CHAPTER 1 – WHAT THE OTHER DETOX PROGRAMS PROMISE

Do you wake up one day and discovered that you are overweight? Impossible! Being overweight is also a process.

Read: it didn't happen overnight? So, don't expect quick fixes or results. You cannot expect to 'detox' in a day and have maximum results.

If you are planning to undergo a 1-day or 7-day detox, then do not expect maximum and long-lasting effects. Granted, there might be some minor changes to your body. However, there are also dangers to losing weight using a diet that entails very low caloric intake. Danger ahead!

These are actually the diet plans that are doomed to fail sooner or later. Eventually, you'll find yourself doing most of your old eating habits again in just a week or two.

There's a CYCLE here: failure leads to depression, depression leads to binging, binging leads to more depression and depression then leads to negative thoughts and perceptions, thinking that you will never achieve the body that you always wanted. EVER!

Afterwards, when a new diet plan is introduced in the market, you'll jump into the bandwagon and the cycle will start anew. And the ending? More depression than what it is when you first tried the diet plan! Believe me, I know how this vicious cycle works. Been there, done that.

The majority of the youngsters reading my book (Thank you!) will disagree with me that any 7-day detox diets will never make you wear that sexy dress by next weekend or so. It might have or it might be. The reason behind this is that younger bodies have the ability to bounce back really quickly than that of the older folks. That's a fact!

Wisdom comes with age. With that, older folks are aware that the more you depend on 7-, 10- or 21-day detox plans, the worse the results will become. An honest piece of advice: youngsters should start to pursue a healthy eating path NOW! [I really should emphasize the word otherwise it'll catch up in due time.]

For youngsters and old folks, I am 100% sure that most of us tried and achieved weight loss goals using a diet or detox plan. The question now is: HOW LONG UNTIL YOU FELL BACK INTO UNHEALTHY EATING HABITS AGAIN? Now, not all of us will answer this question as honestly as we should.

Getting out of the diet mentality isn't easy, but hey it is not impossible either. Don't set yourself up for failure again. You deserve better than this. I will tell you my secret. A more healthful and sustaining diet plan will give you the best results.

I will tell you more about my secret detox diet (that will no longer be a secret once I tell you).

Please understand that what you need right now is someone who will understand your losing weight journey. This unique detox will make you feel good about yourself minus the guilt and depression. It will boost your appearance (yes, I said that) as well as your energy level. It will also increase mental clarity and focus and balance moods. You'll get sick less often and you will have a more positive outlook in life.

A 7-day detox diet cannot do all these, but my unique detox diet program can. I cannot emphasize that weight loss goals must be achieved using a smart detox plan to produce healthy and long-lasting results.

CHAPTER 2 – WHAT THE OPTIMUM APPROACH TO DETOX DIET SHOULD BE

What sets my detox diet apart from other detox programs, you might ask. Simple: HOMEOSTATIS! Homeostasis refers to the ability and tendency of an organism or cell to maintain internal balance as it adjusts the physiological processes thereby compensating the changes in the environment.

A perfect example of homeostasis that we know is our own body's ability to maintain its temperature at 98.6 degrees regardless of the ambient temperature. Our bodies have a tendency to seek, reach and then maintain homeostasis each second we live. As such, our body maintains balance by expending more energy and thus we experience more ramifications.

When it comes to natural detoxification, our body is also amenable as it fixes, reverses and eliminates any issues as well as unnatural factors that it comes in contact with. We breathe, eat, drink and even put some things on our skin. External elements are brought inside our body through these processes.

Essentially, if your food intake is mostly characterized by unhealthy food choices, the body unnecessarily needs to expend more energy in breaking down these wrong foods into absorbable elements. These are 'wrong foods' that contains little nutrients and yet our body should process and send off for our cell's utilization. There are two bad effects of such: 1) our body becomes overworked and 2) our bodies are hindered to reach homeostasis.

That's why WE SHOULD EAT THE RIGHT FOODS! This keeps the balance and maintains a healthy weight.

The science behind homeostasis as a secret to losing weight naturally is factoring in the importance of balance. Our goal is to diet ACCORDINGLY so we can be supportive of the balancing efforts of our body which eventually leads to weight loss and thus a healthier body.

Ignoring balance and the right foods and applying improper weight loss program will only lead to ill health. Oppositely, embracing such a new concept will lead to the most effective and healthiest way of losing weight.

Such a new idea, homeostasis that is, is what sets my unique detox diet to other detox programs out there. My detox diet is:

- Compliant with the principle of alkaline/acid level balance;
- Inclusive of transition diet with helpful tips and hints;
- About optimizing the natural functions of the body;
- About strengthening cells, glands and organs; and
- About the consumption of pure water and wholesome foods.

My detox diet is NOT:

- A miracle or quick-fix strategy;
- About forcing toxins expulsion out of your body; and
- Going to utilize any detox powder, pill or supplement.

Upon learning my detox diet, there might be some issues or concerns on your side especially on the validity of my claims. I expect this. Nonetheless, I highly encourage my readers to conduct their own research to determine the truth behind the claims and learn more about them.

Be reminded that I live and breathe natural health and healing. It is my passion hands down. Through years of experience as a natural health coach, I realized that truths about health have been kept to most of us. Thanks to technology (www and Internet that is), we gain easy access to great knowledge. Untruths are now exposed for the world to discern.

Today, TRUTHS AND UNTRUTHS intermingled online. So, you should be diligent enough to decipher the motives of your sources (and who wrote them). Dig deeper and find true answers.

CHAPTER 3 – SO WHAT'S TRUE DETOX DIET IS...?

I know, I know. The words alkaline and acid might have freaked you out, thinking of your chemistry class where you experiment pH level through litmus papers. What have we learned during those times is that acid is corrosive. It causes severe damage to the skin when touched. So, why would we want acid on our body?

Our body has 100 trillion cells, and these cells produce acid wastes at the cellular level every day of our lives. These wastes must be eliminated or neutralized properly otherwise the body will suffer the consequences. Acid buildups in the body manifest as minor aches or pain such as on the neck and shoulders and skin issues like eczema and acne. Unfortunately, some experience irregular bower movement and weight gain as the manifestation of the buildup.

Further, the accumulation of acids over the years can lead to cancers, stroke, heart problems and lung problems, among other diseases. Acidosis, or the excessive acid accumulation in the body, is often the cause of most health issues.

And the major culprit? The unhealthy foods we eat. Animal products, animal byproducts and grains as well as processed, cooked and fatty foods become acid ash after digestion. In reversing the acid buildup, we must consume healthy alkalizing foods that expedite the task. Apart from this, these foods supply nutrients that assist in rebuilding and regenerating the cells and tissues.

Here's the crux of true detox diet: a healthy eating plan to achieve balance through the consumption of healthy, alkalizing foods. And here's the crux of my detox diet: a healthy eating plan that is physiologically and anatomically designed to be eaten and consumed by the body. With this, the diet can be consumed every day to keep the natural processes in order and maintain a good health throughout.

CHAPTER 4 – WHAT WE ARE REALLY?

Look at your body. What are you – a carnivore, omnivore or herbivore? Well, I don't consider myself as any of these. Instead, I am a FRUGIVORE and so are you.

Frugivorism is the newest archeological finding of the human origin especially in tropical regions where overabundance of fruits is evident. Frugivores differ from fruitarians since they only eat fruits. Frugivores eat fruits (80%), greens (15%) and seeds and nuts (5%). Yes, these are eaten RAW.

You might think that the diet is radically different from what you are accustomed to eating. Let me tell you this. The truth is the diet that you have today is the radical one and not this.

Frugivorism is the original and true diet of the human race until it veered far from it because of many factors. Ultimately, the journey towards becoming omnivorous, carnivorous and herbivorous led to becoming more vulnerable to all kinds of diseases. This is especially true among westernized civilizations without realizing that frugivorism is the epitome of great heath!

What we are witnessing today are people who eat SAD or the standard American diet – a diet that include acid-producing foods. If we only understand what and how acidosis can wreak havoc on your body including major stresses on the systems and organs, you'll drop your SAD diet like a hot potato and choose my detox diet instead to improve your health.

CHAPTER 5 – WHAT YOU DON'T UNDERSTAND ABOUT BODY DETOX

Sadly, there are several misconceptions about body detox in general. Here are some few yet most alarming of these misconceptions.

1) Our body detoxifies itself

Some people think that our body doesn't need any help in detoxifying itself. Actually, it does! It needs external sources to detoxify. However, it doesn't need products that claim to be a natural detox, purging out toxins in the body in a rather harsh manner. What it needs are healthy foods in eliminating toxins naturally and not unnaturally formulated detox products.

When experiencing diseases and discomfort while losing weight, it means that the body is not getting the right tools it needs to balance itself out. My detox diet is ready to provide such tools.

Remember that our body has various functions. Food is needed to supply us with adequate energy in transpiring these functions. In ingesting foods, our body will work hard in digesting, absorbing, utilizing and eliminating wastes. If our body is not getting the right amount of nutrients, it will biologically transmutate the existing nutrients into other nutrients needed by it to transpire some functions. Imagine what your body has to go through only because you are not eating healthily.

We can never underestimate what our body can do. However, if you continue eating low-nutrient foods, it will eventually take a toll on our body through physical stresses. These stresses are detrimental to our health and wellbeing. You will feel bloated or constipated due to acid buildup. This will not happen if you consume foods with alkalizing properties as they help the body to continuously function and detox naturally.

Most of you may argue that you are a not-so-healthy eating plan for several years and you haven't experienced any health issue. Not true. If you are really healthy as you might think then why drink coffee to ward off the grogginess. Also, do you always jump out of your bed with adequate energy to get you through the day? Do you even sleep soundly? If you don't, then these are the effects of poor eating habit that should be changed sooner than later.

2) Detoxification is only possible through purging

Most people think that detoxification is designed to remove toxins by "cleansing." While elimination is an important part of detoxification, there should be more to it. When I say more, I mean that the body must be aided to function normally at its best and on its own.

So, okay, detoxifying the body through taking detox pills or drinking detox juice gets the job of cleansing the body. However, it only subjects the body to more damaging effects in the future. For instance, if you are taking detox products that usually contain laxative, this can disable the peristaltic action of the bowel and it will become more dependent on laxative for movement.

My detox diet will not do this. Instead, it will help your body in reversing acids and thereby eliminating toxins. The detox diet will also help in the proliferation of healthy cells. This also strengthens the cells for the body to function more optimally.

When toxins are removed, and so are parasites. Parasites, which are mostly microscopic, live inside our body. They do have a purpose, however, and that is cleaning up dead organisms. In fact, parasites are considered as the major janitors in the world. We can perceive them as good because of their purpose.

Essentially, if we will cut off the food supply of these decayed and decaying cells because of acid buildup, we can get rid of these parasites. If we get rid of them in other ways, who will clean up our body? Ideally, we can get rid of parasites by getting rid of the dead cells through alkalizing our body and by means of a detox diet – the frugivore diet, that is. The parasites won't sustain.

However, if bigger, non-microscopic parasites are inside your body, the only way to eliminate them is purging. These must be eliminated immediately, but in a healthy way.

3) Detox diet programs are similar to weight loss programs

The safest and most effective detox diet programs help in balancing out your weight. When we say safe and effective, it means that the detox program must be applicable not only for people who want to lose weight, but also for those who are underweight and want to reach a rather healthy weight.

There are several diet programs that force eaters to eat less and less with each meal and that integrate various weight loss products that only the manufacturers know what are contained in them. UGH! Don't you ever dare to try these weight loss programs. Yes, these are weight loss programs that usually promise to lose the extra pounds as much and as quick as possible.

The intention of a detox diet must not be solely about losing weight, but also obtaining good health. As such, you need waste your time, money and energy on these weight loss programs that only abuses your body.

Alternatively, there are some people who believe that we should be eating meat, dairy and grain in addition to vegetable and fruit. This is what've been inculcated in us since we are young – to eat balanced meals every day. These meals include various items in food groups in right proportions to lose weight and thus be healthy. Not so!

I tell you these so called balanced meals will cause you progressive discomfort and illness in the future. We've been brainwashed for so long now! What a shame! Try my detox diet for six months, and you will be amazed at the results. In just six months….

First off, we need to think creatively especially about what are considered as truths and norms. Only then we can take full responsibility of our health through eating what we should we meant to be eating.

CHAPTER 6 – WHAT WE SHOULD BE EATING

Just follow the guidelines set forth in this detox diet program to achieve success in your weight loss journey while also increasing vitality and improving health. I suggest you READ THE GUIDE COMPLETELY before embarking on the detox diet.

You need to transition into my detox diet definitely. Don't fret because I will explain how and why later in this book. For now, I present to you my detox diet – DIET 54321!

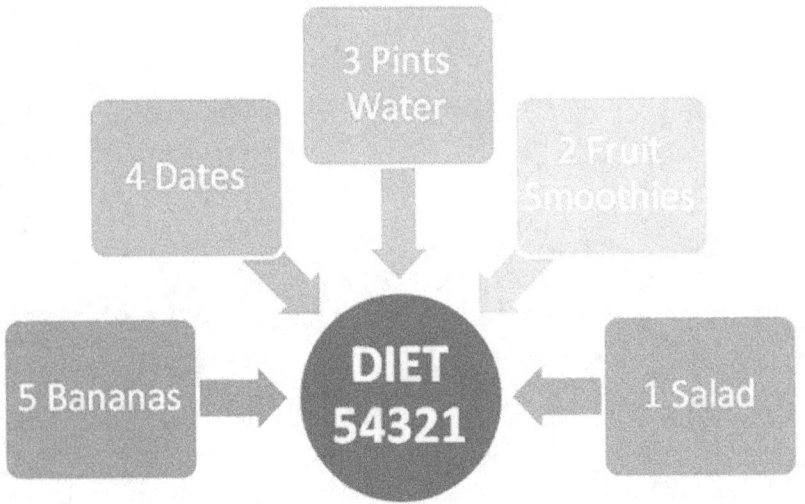

Simple isn't it? The diet may seem drastic at first more so because of what you are accustomed to eating. You may also think that diet 54321 is not sustainable. You might be wondering whether where are the proteins.

Did you know that raw veggies and fruits contain enough amounts of protein in amino acid form? Amazingly, they do! This diet definitely puts healthy eating in a diet program.

The majority of us are too consumed in eating complicated meals with excessive spices, salts, sauces and other ingredients and pairing them with equally unhealthy drinks. It is no wonder then why the westernized countries are plagued with a plethora of digestive problems as well as other major and minor health issues.

Straightforwardly, we eat foods and their combination that we, as humans, should not especially since eating them leads to unnecessary diseases and illnesses. Diet 54321 is a rather simple diet as our body is physically designed to consume them.

The diet is very simple, but not as easy as one might think... at first. As you go along with it, you will notice that your cravings are diminished, energy levels went up and overall health improved. If you are suffering from any skin issues, it will be reversed as well. Really, these are just some of the amazing results of the diet.

Definitely, the essence of the diet is eating based on a diet eating plan and following such a plan every day. Don't worry though because I will give you some pointers for options and modifications until the body gets used to consuming foods that help in natural detoxification.

IMPORTANT: Skipping any part of Diet 54321 is not advisable. Every part is critical in giving the body the caloric energy it needs in reaching and maintaining its balance and thus help the body shed the extra pounds naturally.

5 BANANAS

In the US, Cavendish banana is the most popular. If you will eat other varieties especially the smaller ones, make sure you eat six to seven of them. Each banana must be at least seven inches or the equivalent. You can eat these bananas at one sitting or throughout the day.

Did you know that banana is considered as the 'nature's perfect food'? Why not? Bananas have nutritive compositions and proportions that mimic just the right types and amounts of nutritional elements that our body requires to keep it healthy. I know some local athletes that lived on eating 30

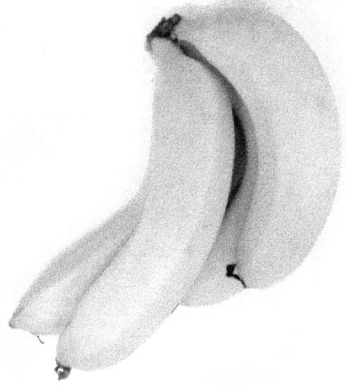

bananas every day. Bizarre but true.

On the other hand, I also know at least three people who dislike the taste of banana. I wonder why because bananas are one of my all time favorite. In fact, bananas are my comfort food. For those people who also do not like bananas (I pity you), I got you covered. For those who enjoy eating bananas….

Remember to eat ripe bananas only. It is very easy to discern ripe from unripe bananas. Unripe bananas are usually green and yellow in color particularly near the stem. Avoid these bananas since they are highly acidic. If you must, buy about three to five bunches of bananas a few days before you begin this diet. The premise is buy bananas so they'll get ripe and ready to be consumed in a few days.

Tip: Keep the bananas closer together, so they'll ripen faster than expected. If the bananas tend to ripen too fast and you won't be eating them in a few days, just take the ripened bananas apart from the rest. Put them in a separate basket, for instance, and the ripening process will be slowed down.

Alternatively, you may put the ripened bananas on the fridge to delay ripening. Frozen bananas are very good for smoothies.

If you don't like to eat bananas, eat substitutes. While my detox diet is not based on calorie counts, I advise that you eat fruit substitutes of about 500 calories. You may refer to online calorie calculators to help you with this. Here are some of my suggestions to one banana replacement.

1 big apple
1 ¼ cups of blueberries
2 medium (or 3 small) oranges
2 cups of cubed cantaloupe

In substituting the five bananas, you may eat a variety of fruits day by day. For example, you may eat 1 big apple today, 2 medium oranges the next day, 3 bananas and 1 medium orange the day after that, etc. Also, you may eat 1 banana in the morning, 1 cup of cubed cantaloupe in the afternoon and ¾ cups of blueberries in the evening. This is just a matter of preference, mind you.

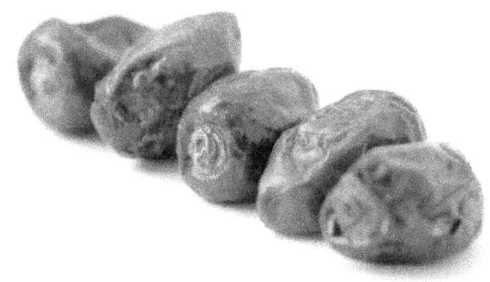

4 DATES

I love Medjool dates! They are really hard to resist. Dates must be included in the diet as a substitute for sweets (and junk food). Delectable as they are, dates are like your favorite caramel candy only that dates are healthier. Not all fruits are sweet enough to satisfy our sweet tooth, so surely, dates can do the trick.

The best part is dates can be included in raw desserts to make them healthier. For example, you may mash dates with a pinch of carob power. Then, layer with 1/4-inch thick sliced bananas. What a treat! You may eat this dessert guilt-free.

Originally, dates are considered as one of the weight loss foods. They can keep the body full, so you don't have to reach for sweet junk foods whenever you feel the craving for them. Dates are rich in fiber which helps in regular bowel movement.

When buying date, read the labels in packaging for the dried fruits. Make sure that there are no sulfites (or sulphates) in the list of ingredients. Medjool dates are available commercially. Walmart sells them, and so are other major grocery chains. Check both the dried fruits and produce sections when looking for dates.

There are many types of dates, but Medjool is the most popular of them all. Eat larger-sized dates. However, if you can find the smaller ones, eat more to satisfy the diet requirement.

Tip: If the dates are dried or not plump enough, soak them in water for up to one hour (if needed) before eating or blending them.

3 PINTS WATER

Any health regime is not complete without emphasizing the need to drink at least eight glasses of water every day. Water not only replenishes and quenches our thirst, but it also helps in flushing the toxins out of our body.

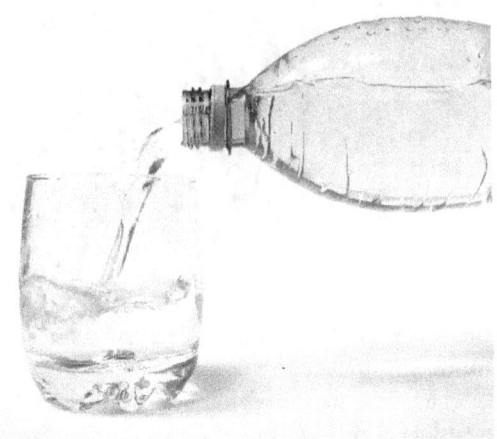

Did you know that 72% of our body is water? Of course, you know that. We perspire and urinate and thus we lost water. To keep the water in our body at that level, we must replenish to compensate what we've lost due various processes inside our bodies. Water keeps our body hydrated!

Let's go back to eight glasses of water that what've thought to drink on a daily basis. Roughly, eight glasses are equivalent 64 ounces of water. I was thought before that the water consumption must depend on how active you are and your weight. If you are a not very active person, divide your weight in pounds by two and that's how many ounces of water you should drink. If you are active, you should drink 2/3 ounces of water.

So, if you are not active and you weigh 200 pounds, you must be drinking 100 ounces of water (approximately 13 glasses of water). If you are active and you weigh 200 pounds, you should drink 133 ounces of water (approximately 17 glasses of water). Whoa!

This alone makes me cringe. Do you force yourself to drink water and feel bloated in the end? I always think that there is something so ambiguous with drinking that amount of water or so I thought. The question now is what's the right amount of water that we must drink or is there really such a thing - right amount of water?

This is the reason why I include [AT LEAST] three pints water in my detox diet. Inside our body is too much acidity, and water, calcium and cholesterol are need components to lessen the acidity within. Acidity is the reason why we feel dehydrated.

Drinking at least three pints water every day in addition to the water contents in the fruits will make your body hold on to the water that's giving you a bloated feeling.

Bloating is a sign that your body is acidic, but this will soon be over once you get used to drinking lots of water. If possible, drink pure or home-distilled water. Fresh spring water will also do.

As the body draws near to reaching balance, which means that the acid in your body is becoming neutralized, you will eventually need to decrease the amount of your water intake. In the end, you might have to drink water only when you are thirsty.

Along with water, veggies and fruits also contain water that helps in rehydrating the body. All of these contain nutrients, electrolytes and alkalizing properties that our body needs in fending off acids and maintaining its healthy condition. This only means that if you will stop the Diet 54321 and go back to your most meat, dairy, grain and fat diet, acidosis may also return and you will feel more dehydrated again.

Digging deeper into electrolytes, perhaps you have heard (and drank) Powerade or Gatorade to replenish your body. Don't believe the ads too much because these drinks have high acidity levels. Gatorade, for instance, has a pH level of 3 wherein the neutral number is 7. Don't depend on these drinks because they can lead to further acidosis and dehydration.

2 FRUIT SMOOTHIES

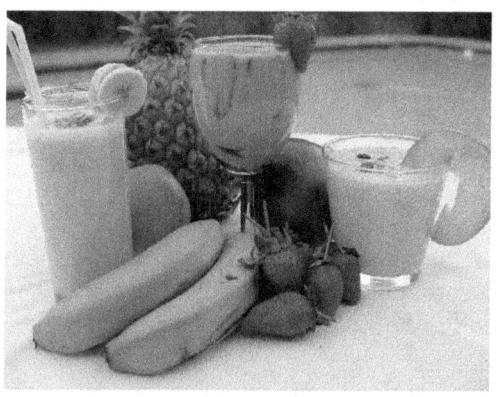

Additional caloric requirements are attainable through having some smoothies, but of course, these should be healthy. For men and active women, they require more calories on a daily basis. Their smoothies must be 40 ounces at the very least. For smaller built individuals, at least 30 ounces of smoothies are enough.

Smoothies are everywhere thus there's no need to think of where to get them, that is, if you cannot do them at home. Smoothies are a great way to replenish the lost hydration and nutrients especially after a physically-exhausting workout.

As much as possible, go for a fruit smoothie. They taste good and are highly nutritious. In fact, you can consider a fruit smoothie as a full meal. Smoothies are very easy to make and anyone in the family can enjoy them. For the most appealing smoothies for you, choose your favorite fruit(s).

Tip: Invest in a high quality blender. Quality determines the variation that the blender can process and how well the foods are processed. Fundamentally, high quality blenders have longer lifespan and warranty.

The majority of the residents today have a blender that can be used in concocting the best smoothies. Honestly though, the average blender that you have right now may not be the perfect blender for this detox diet.

Average blenders cannot produce the right consistency of a smoothie. They didn't blend enough, but if you prefer smaller chunks of fruits to go with your smoothie, average blenders are just fine.

Just make sure that your average blender can do the job for you if you opt to use it anyway otherwise you will have to purchase a new blender every three months or less. If you have the money to burn (along with your calories, pun intended), then invest on a high-durable and high-speed blender.

If you haven't made your own smoothie before, don't worry because it's easy-peasy. You are going to need a liquid base like water, freshly-made juice or fresh coconut milk. Make sure that the juice or coco milk is fresh and is not store-brought. The amount of the liquid base will determine the thickness of your smoothie. Experiment on this.

For the fruits, the healthiest options are organic, seasonal, local and harvested-ripe fruits. Good for you if you have organically-grown fruits on your backyard or if you have immediate access to a farmer's market. If not, the best option is visiting the fresh produce sections of your favorite grocery store. Some grocery stores have a selection of frozen organic fruits that still have all the nutrients in them.

Throw in some sliced avocado or banana to make the smoothie creamier. To make it sweeter, add organic yet nutritious sweeteners such as yacon root, stevia, agave nectar, maple syrup or honey. As for me, I just use Medjool dates to make my smoothie sweeter.

If you want to make a 'green' smoothie, throw in some leafy greens into the blender. This also helps in consuming the right amount of greens in your daily diet. Just blend them in and no other people will know what's in them. Not even your kids!

You can use any type of fruits, but don't you ever add unhealthy, acidic options such as:

- Unripe fruits
- Green, unripe bananas
- Cranberries
- Prunes
- Sulphured dried fruits

If you don't want a smoothie, you may replace it with its fruit equivalent. Think of the amount of the fruit that you will be putting onto your smoothie. This is the amount of fruits that you should be eating as a replacement to the smoothie.

If you prefer juice, this is also acceptable. However, I do not suggest replacing smoothies with juices often because the latter are usually less filling and they are low in fiber.

If eventually you reach your weight loss goal (which you will), you may try drinking grape juice. I call this grape juice fasting wherein I drink grape juice for two to five days after two to three weeks of making and drinking smoothies. Before you embark on a juice fast, however, you should be doing Diet 54321 for at least 2 months to ensure that your body will accommodate the juice fast.

1 SALAD

Salads must be composed of ¾ to a pound of greens. Greens that should go into your salad must include lettuces except iceberg lettuce, arugula, spinach, parsley, kale, beet greens, dandelion greens, collard greens and Swiss chard. Salads must be in big serving bowls the way I like mine.

You may eat the greens alone or you can add toppings such as carrot, celery, sweet corn, bell peppers, sprouts, beet, cucumber, zucchini, tomato, squash, scallion, asparagus or cabbage. Regardless of your choice(s), they must be raw!

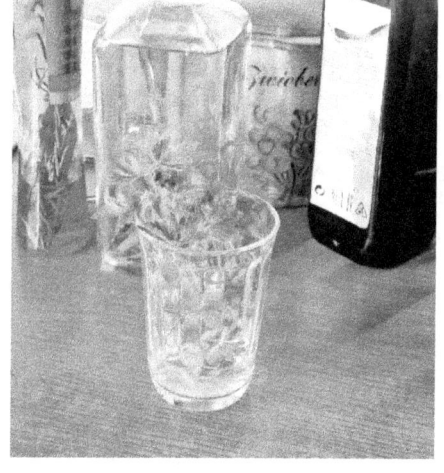

You may also add in fruits like apple, orange or pineapple. If you are suffering from arthritis or any inflammatory condition, avoid eating cruciferous veggies. Some examples are kale, arugula, cauliflower, broccoli and cabbage although you may browse online for a complete list cruciferous veggies.

Tip: Eat the salad as your last meal of the day. High energy fruits won't help in trying to sleep fast, but the salad will ground your energy. When eating salads, chew the foods well before swallowing them, greens are difficult to digest than fruits. Remember that digestion starts in our mouth.

When preparing salads, think about your own convenience. You need not spend the whole day on your kitchen every single day. Make up to four or five salads at a time and store them on a Ziploc bag. Don't forget to push out the air inside the bags, reducing unwanted oxidation in the process. Also, make more raw salad dressings to go with your salad. Dressings' lifespan is expected to be between three to four days wherein the nutrients remain intact.

Never whipped your own salad dressing before? Here are some recipes that you may try:

Orange-Mango Dresing
- 1 cup diced mango
- 1 small or medium orange
- 3 to 4 pcs. Medjool dates
- 2 tbsp. raw cashews or other nuts/seeds
- a quarter-sized ginger root
- 1/8 to 1/4 cup water
- 1/4 cup scallion (optional
-

Avocado-Orange Dressing
- 1/2 avocado
- 1 large orange
- 1/2 large bell pepper (red, orange or yelow)
- 3 scallions or
- 1 garlic clove

Zucchini-Avocado Dressing
- 1 small chopped zucchini
- 1/2 small avocado
- 2 tbsps walnuts or raw pine nuts
- 1 to 1 1/2 lemon juice
- 1/2 tbsps fresh dill
- 1 small pinch chives
- 1/2 clove garlic

You need not skimp on using these dressings. There are thousands of dressing recipes online that you can collect, print and follow. When it comes to YOUR salad, eat anything you like.

If preparation time was a problem, you might as well stock some ingredients of easy-to-whip dressing. Make sure you have lemons or limes on the fridge. Lemon juice on a salad is actually one of the healthiest dressing choices. If you want sweet and sour, add honey, agave nectar or stevia. If you don't want lemons, then choose orange. Squeeze the orange on your salad and sprinkle it with some dill, chives or parsley. These are simple salad dressings yet are very satisfying.

For salad variations, you may purchase a tri-blade vegetable cutter (or spiralizer) that cuts veggies in spiral, shoestring, pasta-like or noodle-like cuts. With this, you can make your own zucchini noodles. Just spiralize abut two to four small to medium zucchinis and then add any of the salad dressing of your choice. Or, you can try my raw spaghetti sauce recipe below.

Raw Spaghetti Sauce
Blend:

- 2 to 3 cups of Cherry or Roma tomatoes
- 1/2 large mango
- 1/2 cup bell pepper
- 1/4 cup all-natural, sun-dried tomatoes
- 3/4 chopped celery
- 2 tbsps fresh basil
- 1/2 tbsps fresh oregano

CHAPTER 7 – ARE THERE ANY ALLOWABLE FATS?

Yes! Fats generally vary. Basically, there are good and bad fats. Animal fats, as well as dairies and meats, must be avoided totally. Instead, you may choose and eat plant-based fats that tend to be healthier. Just DON'T OVERDO IT.

I don't want you to count your fat intake. That's absurd. However, what I will give you is a 'safe fats list' that you may incorporate in your smoothie, salad or dressing. Here are the safe fats I am talking about:

- ½ cup raw seeds and nuts
- 1/3 medium avocado
- 20 medium olives
- 1 tbsp organic olive oil
- 1 tbsp coconut oil

9 CHAPTER 8 – ARE THERE ANY EXCEPTIONS OR SUBSTITUTIONS?

We cannot control all the circumstances around us. So, I figure there should be some exceptions and substitutions when the need for such arises.

For salad dressings, you may instead by bottled dressings, but make sure they are all-natural. Ensure that there are no dairies in the ingredients. Follow the instructions in storing the bottled dressing to keep its freshness.

When you are out with your loved ones or friends, you might veer slightly away from this detox diet. Certainly, eat something healthy otherwise your blood sugar will go too low. If you are at a friend's house, you may munch on veggies like carrots if there are no fruits. Whatever you do or wherever you are, don't make yourself go hungry.

If it is possible, bring your fruits, smoothie and salad with you if you are traveling. Put them in a cooler to keep them cool and fresh. If it is an unplanned trip or visit, always choose the smartest [and healthiest] choice so you don't have to skip eating.

Finally, you may drink hot or cold natural herbal teas. The teas shouldn't contain any caffeine though.

CHAPTER 9 – WILL I EXPERIENCE ANY ADVERSE SYMPTOMS OR EFFECTS?

Before I teach you how to transition to Diet 54321 properly, let me tell you about the detox symptoms or detox effects. It is your right to know all about this.

We feel these effects or symptoms on our body, and they manifest in various forms. Sometimes, especially on the early stages, you may feel sick. You may suffer from headache, nausea, dizziness, diarrhea, fever, etc. You may also feel skin eruptions such as acne and rashes. The healthcare professionals consider these manifestations as a diseases or sickness which they will try to suppress and heal.

Realistically though, inside your body are several issues that are currently taking place. The body will reverse or eliminate these issues through trying to detoxify itself. The natural detox processes are these manifestations.

Some people believe that the existence of any of these illnesses is a major problem. Wrong! These are our body's natural reaction to the changes that we subject our bodies to. Our body is actually getting rid of the problem experienced by balancing itself through detoxification.

So what's the correlation between eating healthy and feeling the symptoms, you might ask. Simply, when your body starts to reverse acidosis, which is the problem, it will begin feeling the repercussions in the form of sickness.

Bottom-line, LISTEN TO YOUR BODY! In the event that the detox diet becomes too harsh for you, you may instead choose any of the cheaties that I listed below. Don't munch of other foods other than the ones listed here, so no meats, grains or dairies.

CHAPTER 10 – WHAT ARE THE CHEATIES AVAILABLE?

There are instances that you may crave for cooked meals. Personally, I strongly believe that it is always better to give in than to fight the cravings.

You may choose to store some cheaties that you can reach for whenever there is a craving for junk food. However, I don't mean the junk food that you used to eat. What I mean is the healthier version of junk food if there is such a thing. These cheaties had helped me while I am transitioning, but don't abuse them.

These cheaties will not only help you during episodes of craving, but they will also fend off the detox symptoms more so when they get too difficult to handle. They can actually slow down the natural detox processes. Here they are:

1) Veggie soup or steamed veggies – Make a large batch, put them in serving-sized containers and keep them in the fridge. The veggies must not be overcooked.

2) Baked sweet potatoes – Make one small or medium or ½ large sweet potato. Eat it plain (without cream or butter). Do not microwave the sweet potato.

3) Organic brown rice – Cook it like your favorite plain rice. Basmati rice is very healthy.

4) Millet bread – Reach for a piece whenever you feel the urge. Millet bread is healthy because it's gluten-free.

5) Air-popped popcorn – Prepare your popcorn as is without salt. Microwaving popcorn is acceptable.

6) Xochitl (pronounced as ozchill) – This is corn chips brand, but it is very healthy since it is all-natural and gluten-free. It is also dairy-free, wheat-

free, no preservatives and no trans fat.

CHAPTER 11 – IS EXERCISING REQUIRED?

I cannot emphasize it enough that, for acidic individuals, downtime may be required from time to time while transitioning. You should heed to such need. Again, you must LISTEN TO YOUR BODY.

There are certain days when you feel like resting the whole day. It is okay. If you can, you may do brisk walking or biking at a slow speed. You may also do light house chores. If you are working out regularly, you should forgo weightlifting. You may also do some yoga, but limit it to low-powered exercises such as passive stretches.

The bottom-line is save more energy so your body will get back to its balance quicker. Thus, if your body wants to rest, then do so.

CHAPTER 12 – HOW SHOULD I TRANSITION TO THE DIET 54321?

Jumping from SAD to Diet 54321 is rather suicide. My detox diet includes raw, fresh, nutrient-dense and whole food items that may have negative effects emotionally, physically and mentally. For one, the body will be shocked after years of eating meats, dairies and grains.

To minimize the detox symptoms, you must transition properly. This doesn't mean, however, that there won't be any detox effects. These are inevitable, but you can always control them instead of them having control over you and your daily life.

I got you covered. Here's a transition diet plan that may help you to transition gradually from being an unhealthy to a healthy eater. There are actually four transitioning stages, with which each stage requires at least two weeks depending on the acidity level of your body. You can possibly shorten each stage to one week or 10 days, but listening to your body is a must to determine how well it is coping with the adjustments.

Remember that if you go too fast with the diet, you will likely to experience harsher detox effects. If you want, you may escalate each stage up to 4 weeks.

1st Stage:

First meal: Eat fruit(s). Eat until you are full. I am not talking about 1 apple or orange. I mean eat five apples or more or until you are content whatever will fill you up comfortably. If you are in a hurry, prepare a fruit smoothie instead and put it in a carry-anywhere tumbler. Alternatively, you may prepare the smoothie the night before if you are going to leave the house early in the morning. Don't make any excuses more so because adjustments will take some time. Just avoid relying on grabbing leftovers or buying fast foods.

Snack time: Eat a fruit snack between each meals especially when you are feeling sluggish. You may eat ripe bananas until you are full. If you prefer sweets, just eat five to ten Medjool dates. Go and grab any fruit that you want. Since you are still eating meats, dairies and grains as part of your major meals, eat fruits one hour before a major meal and two hours after.

Veggie salad: During lunch or dinner, eat a large bowl of veggie salad. I mean the salad should be your main course and the rest as your side dish. Better yet, eat the salad alone as the entire meal if you are used to eating such.

Avoid dairy: Check the package of anything packed that you will eat. Read the list of ingredients. Dairy products are hidden in various forms. Dairies are our worst enemies in lieu with eating healthy. Perhaps, you should Google the term "milk myth" so you'd understand what I'm saying. Dairies are not only the cause of high acidity in our bodies, they also cause congestion.

You should be eating what you are normally eating in addition to the foods I outlined above. You simply have to add fruits and salads and get rid of dairies.

2nd Stage:

At this stage, continue doing the first stage and then add the following elements.

No meat: Perhaps, you don't know this but our body needs no protein. Our body cannot use such unless the protein is broken down into amino acids. It is in the form of amino acids that protein can be absorbed and utilized by the body. However, breaking down proteins requires nutrients and energy.

Basically, animal products are high in protein. They are also acidic, next to dairies. Replace meat with brown rice or baked sweet potato. These are as filling as meats.

A serving of starch: Eat starch such as breads and pastas. You may also eat white rice or white potato.

Cheats: Start to incorporate any of the cheaties that I listed.

3rd Stage:

Again, at this stage, continue doing the first two stages while adding the following elements.

Veggie meals: During lunch and dinner, eat steamed veggies and salad. The salad can be a mix of different veggie and greens or a particular green if you want. The steamed veggies can be replaced with brown rice, baked sweet potato or vegan soup, whatever you desire.

Avoid salt and fat: Salt is pretty self-explanatory although it is okay to have a little fat on your salad dressing.

4th Stage:

If the grocery store is not carrying ripe bananas, you might as well purchase the unripe ones. However, make sure you purchase one week before starting the detox diet. Just remember that if you are doing the first stage for two weeks, the succeeding stages must be also two weeks each.

1st week:

On days 1, 4 and 7, follow the diet.

On days, 2, 3, 5 and 6, these are your off days. Eat fruit or a smoothie on your first meal. Eat only two small or one large salad, steamed veggie (or vegan soup) and fruits for the rest of the day. Eat lots of a variety of fruits.

If this sounds slightly difficult for you, follow the diet plan on day 1 and then consider days 2, 4 and 6 as the days off. If you are comfortable with this enough, you may add two more days to your days on diet (days 1, 4 and 7) and one more day to your days off diet (days 2 to 3 and days 5 to 6).

This is the reason why I tell you that you cannot go too fast and transition gradually by alternating the number of weeks required in each stage. This will all depend on your preferences and adjustments. The 2-week rule is not a hard rule, just a guideline.

2nd week:

In this week, alternate the days on and days off diet. For instance, you may choose days 9, 11 and 13 as your days on diet and choose days 8, 10 and 12 as your days off diet, if we will continue the 1st week above.

Further, here are some daily menu examples once you have transitioned successfully to Diet 54321. Remember that while you may have fruit smoothies, it is critical that follow the 5, 4, 3, 2 and 1 requirement of intake. You can alternate the first 4, but the salad MUST BE EATEN LAST.

1st day:
Eat the first smoothie as your first meal.
After 2 hours, eat 3 bananas.
During lunch, eat 2 bananas and 2 dates.
At snack time, eat 2 dates.
After 2 to 3 hours, eat the second smoothie.
Finally, eat a big bowl of salad.
2nd day:
Eat 4 bananas as your first meal.
After 2 to 3 hours, eat 1 banana and 2 dates.
At lunchtime, eat your first smoothie.
During snack time, munch on 2 dates.
Drink your second smoothie.
At dinner, have your salad.
And so on…

If you are working, you can take the fruits, dates and smoothies to work. Store them properly though. Prepare them the night before so you won't be in a hurry the next morning.

CONCLUSION

You should be seeing some results as you go along with following the diet. If while following Diet 54321 and there are no results whatsoever, there could be other reasons why you are not losing weight. These reasons could be physiological or psychological in nature. This only means that your body requires further internal fixing that's why there are no apparent results.

In terms of survival, our body will fix the most critical issues first to balance them out before embarking on and accomplishing other things such as losing weight. Diet 54321 is not about eliminating calories, counting carbs, watching fats, etc. This diet is actually a body balancing diet. Don't give up. It'll happen eventually.

Now, you might be wondering how long Diet 54321 will lead to reaching your desired weight. The answer generally varies as it mostly depends on your own body's imbalances and other health issues. Not even I can say how long will it take for your body to reach a balance. I can only guarantee that you will be at a better state physically, emotionally, mentally when you start shedding the extra pounds. It's cloud nine definitely!

With that, I wish you the best of luck. HAPPY DETOX DIETING WITH MY DIET 54321!

Finally, if you enjoyed this book, please take the time to share your thoughts and post a review on Amazon. It'd be greatly appreciated!

Thank you and good luck!

ABOUT THE AUTHOR

Eric Warren is a practicing Naturopath specializing in healing through nutrition. Along with being a natural health coach, He has also a published author.

Eric has recently published his natural health methods "Super Detox Diet For Weight Loss: Optimize Your Body's Natural Functions To Detox & Cleanse your body, Boost your healt and Loss weight Naturally."

His ultimate goal is to educate as many people as possible about the natural alternative methods , healing powers of food and how to easily incorporate these changes into daily life.